The R
(and

MW00848637

"A really effective guide! My wife is now very very happy."
— *Brett, 35, Indianapolis*

"My fiancé and I enjoyed reading this together. Now we're more open and comfortable expressing what we want."
— *Charlene, 32, Las Vegas*

"Excellent! I thought my wife's feedback kept me up on the art of pleasure. Now I've got many new techniques I am excited to try."
— *Larry, 48, Key West*

"As always, Dr. Sadie rocked it again! Love that her books are easy to read and full of fantastic information!"
— *Sarah, 52, Houston*

"A must read. No one is born good at sex, and just like anything you get good at, you need to learn and practice. This book gives you the learning—the practice is up to you!"
— *Ken, 22, Newark*

"Very well written. I learned a lot and now I'm anxious to put my newfound knowledge to good use. The illustrations are tasteful and informative."
— *Joseph, 33, Minneapolis*

"Something FINALLY helped my hubby understand my body! **Woo-hoo!** Now we know what triggers and activates...and how to amp it up!"
— *Catherine, 41, San Francisco*

"Dr. Sadie has a gift for showing guys like me what a woman wants. That's a doctor's appointment I'll always race to!"
— *Jay, 47, New York*

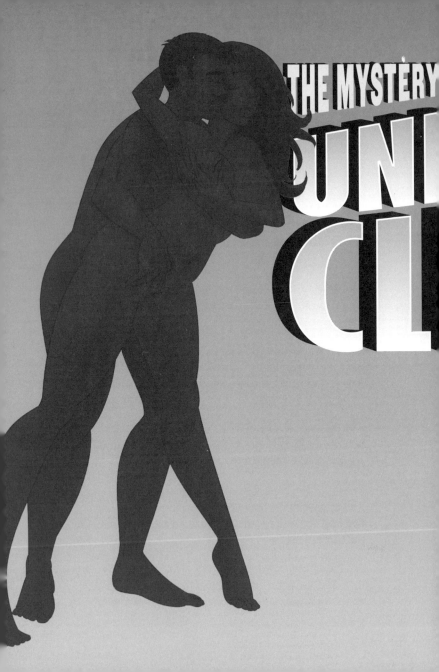

THE SUPERCOVER TORIS

ORGASMIC FINGERTIP TOUCHING EVERY WOMAN CRAVES — ILLUSTRATED

DR. SADIE ALLISON

ILLUSTRATED BY ANDREW WISLOCKI

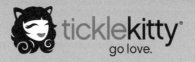

ticklekitty®
go love.

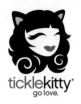

ticklekitty®
go love.

Tickle Kitty, Inc.
San Francisco, CA U.S.A.
Fax: (415) 876-1900
TickleKitty.com

The Mystery of the Undercover Clitoris
Orgasmic Fingertip Touching Every Woman Craves

Author: Dr. Sadie Allison
Editor: J. Crocker Norge
Cover Art & Illustrator: Andrew Wislocki
Cover Design: Meat and Potatoes, Inc.
Layout: Daniel Chan Design
Author Photos: Vance Jacobs

Copyright © 2014–2015 by Tickle Kitty, Inc. All rights reserved.
ISBN: 978-0-9914914-0-7
Printed in the U.S.A.

PLEASE NOTE
This book is intended for educational and entertainment purposes only.
Neither the Author, Illustrator, nor Publisher is responsible for the use or
misuse of any sexual techniques discussed here, or for any loss, damage,
injury or ailment caused by reliance on any information contained in this
book. Please use common sense. The illustrations in this book depict
couples who are in faithful, monogamous relationships. Readers who are not
monogamous, or who have not been tested for STIs (sexually transmitted
infections) are strongly urged to employ the safer sex practices in Chapter 9.
If you have any health issues or other concerns, you should consult a qualified
healthcare professional or licensed therapist *before* trying any techniques.

ADD TO YOUR COLLECTION & ADD TO YOUR
Satisfaction

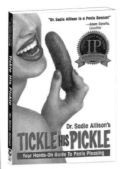

Tickle His Pickle
Your Hands-On Guide
to Penis Pleasing

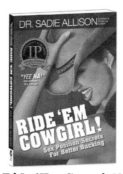

Ride 'Em Cowgirl!
Sex Position Secrets
for Better Bucking

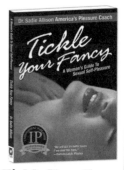

Tickle Your Fancy
A Woman's Guide to
Sexual Self-Pleasure

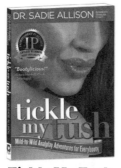

Tickle My Tush
Mild-to-Wild Analplay
Adventures for
Everybooty

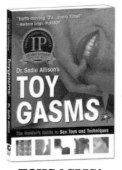

TOYGASMS!
The Insider's Guide
to Sex Toys and
Techniques

Here's to you, *for choosing to be a more thoughtful, generous, world-class lover.*

Inside

10 Thrilling Chapters to Pleasing the Undercover Clitoris

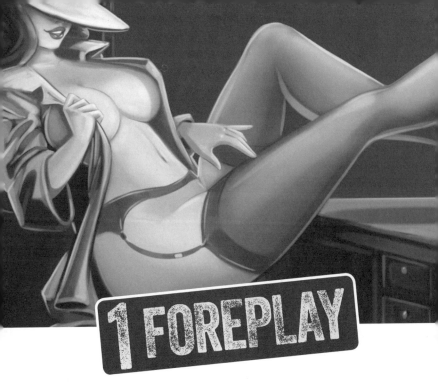

1 FOREPLAY

May I ask a small favor? Place this book on your lap, or on the table in front of you, and turn your palms toward you. Now look carefully at the tips of your fingers.

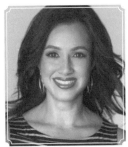

**Dr. Sadie Allison,
America's Pleasure Coach**

Here's my promise to you…

You will never again see your ten digits as mere

1

fingertips. By the time you finish my book, you'll be thinking of them as the most nimble, knowing, living, lively, flexy sex toys womankind has ever experienced.

Okay, you can stop gazing now. It's nearly time for your wife or your girlfriend (or girlfriends!) to begin admiring your fingertips—the instant you can show how much pure orgasmic magic they contain. Even better, you'll soon find your virtuoso performance will inspire her to *return* all that pleasure with equal or greater gusto, since that's what happens when caring, sharing lovers get their libidos in sync.

If that's what you want, welcome! Your sex life is about to experience a lifelong upgrade to Cloud 9.

But first, full disclosure: I possess no mystical powers to bestow on your digits. I am an award-winning Pleasure Coach (as well as a proud Clitoral-American!), here to open up the "other team's playbook" for you, and reveal the many ways your lover PRAYS you'll touch her on the most erotic, exotic, exciting, thrilling wonder spot of her entire naked body.

Her clitoris.

Together, you and I will solve mankind's greatest mystery of "The Undercover Clitoris," because, after all, there really is no mystery at all.

How Have YOUR Lovers Rated You (Secretly)?

While talking recently with some of my closest girlfriends, the subject came up about all the lovers we've had throughout the years—men of all ages, sizes and backgrounds. Each of us had to admit that we really only found one or two with true magic in their fingertips. Sadly, we had to agree that magicians like these are a rare breed. We laughed about how even the most boastful guys proved to be all thumbs below the waist, or worse, chose to completely ignore the clitoris—selfishly barging past any kind of excitement and foreplay directly to The Dry Plunge.

Guess how much unlubricated heat my girlfriends admitted these selfish lovers got in return?

Later that night on the drive home, I decided

that in most cases, it wasn't their fault. No one ever showed these guys how a woman loves her clitoris to be touched. Or they unwisely let porn be their teacher. Or they heard previous lovers utter ill-informed or even ill-advised words. Or their eager hands were continually pushed away by timid lovers.

No wonder these overheated guys knew little about a woman's body! They had no treasure map. No GPS. And no Siri blurting, *"SOFTER!... SLOOOOWER!"*

Early on, before I became a full-time pleasure coach, I found that many guys were truly willing to learn, when I took the time to make discovery fun. That's when it dawned on me that I had a knack for sexual guiding, without bruising their egos or causing embarrassment. Even guys with a few good moves were always eager to learn a few new ones, and I was more than happy to show them.

My point is, clitoral touching is an art. And you, my friend, are about to become Da Vinci.

The Clitoral Playbook (That You've Never Seen)

Since 2001, I've written, published and sold over two million award-winning sex-help books. In the process, my field of view expanded to include all types of people of all ages, granting me a rare and valuable perspective of hetero-sexual mating habits today.

And yet, with all this diversity, one simple truism stands tall:

If a guy speaks clitoris, the world is his oyster.

As you delve deeper inside this book, you'll see exactly why the clitoris is the universal button to your lover's orgasm and passion. (And if it was as easy to operate as an elevator button, you wouldn't need to read this!)

I'll first give you an exciting guided anatomy tour of the entire vulva, so when you part your lover's lips, you won't feel like a newcomer in town.

In Chapter 3, I'll clue you in to the magic elixir called lubrication that activates every one of your lover's millions of pleasure receptors instantly!

Chapter 4 will enlighten you about what happens when your woman comes, and how to amp up those orgasms beyond anything she's ever experienced.

After that, in Chapter 5, you'll find out how and when your lover's sexual stimulation should begin. (*Hint:* It doesn't start the instant your fly unzips.)

In Chapters 6 and 7, I'll provide easy-to-follow advice and close-up views on how you can touch your lover's clitoris. I guarantee you'll want to try these right away (and so will your lover!)

Chapter 8 will offer you unique and comfortable ways to position your bodies so you can maximize the touching pleasures you give to her.

Lastly, I'll wrap up your lesson with a concise guide to what you need to know about safer sex.

(♥)

Enough with the Sermon. Let's Get to the Sex!

I'd like you to keep this thought with you as we explore a woman's most intimate pleasure: *Think of yourself as an expert safecracker.*

To get inside, you must listen carefully. You must feel for subtle changes. You must know the anatomy. And you must engage that sixth sense to tell you when you're closing in.

For there are many untold treasures awaiting you once that door opens wide.

Have fun learning and exploring! And if all this inspires you to miss a full day of work or school, and you need to show a doctor's note, feel free to write to me at *doctorsadie@ticklekitty.com!*

Xxxxs & Ohhhhs,

Dr. Sadie
America's Pleasure Coach

What's Your Clitoral IQ?

Let's see where you stand right now, before you dive in. (And no peeking at the answer key at the end of Chapter 9.)

1. Where do you find the clitoris?
   a) Halfway inside the vagina
   b) Atop the inner folds of the vulva
   c) At the tip of the uvula

2. About how big is an average clitoris?
   a) The size of a small pea
   b) The size of a little toe
   c) The size of an un-erect penis

3. What's the correct pronunciation of "clitoris?"
   a) Kli-TOR-us
   b) KLIT-a-ris
   c) Kli-tor-US

4. What's the best way to touch a clitoris?
   a) Hard and fast
   b) Soft and gentle
   c) Around it, indirectly

(♥)

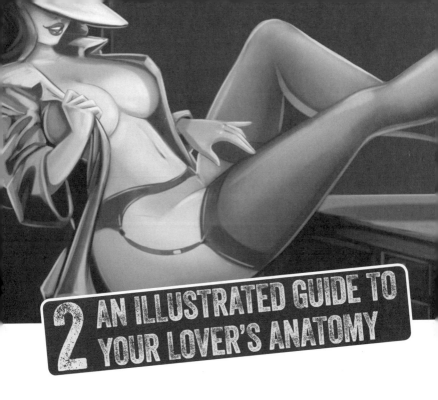

2 AN ILLUSTRATED GUIDE TO YOUR LOVER'S ANATOMY

Even Sherlock Holmes couldn't solve a case without clues. So now that you're here to solve "The Mystery of the Undercover Clitoris," you'd be wise to explore the sensual clues that await within a woman's most delicate setting—a destination that, in all likelihood, you've been calling by the wrong name.

Come Inside the Vulva

Everything you see within your lover's genitals is known as the "vulva." If you're like many guys, you've probably always called it a "vagina," but you'd lose that round to any smart aleck on *Jeopardy*. Here's why: The vulva includes ALL of a woman's external genitalia, while the vagina simply defines the canal where you spend your waking hours planning to plunge your penis!

Why is exploring the entire vulva important? As you'll see, all its joys are interconnected, *especially as your lover nears orgasm*. So understanding her vulva, and how it feels to her to be touched with the brilliance of an artist, lifts you from being a lover who's all-thumbs, to one who gets all thumbs-up.

So welcome to the vulva. Please come inside:

The Lips. Every vulva is wrapped in two sets of lips, an outer pair and an inner pair (labia majora and labia minora, respectively). On the unlikely chance you ever stumbled across photos of various vulvas on the Internet, you

The Vulva

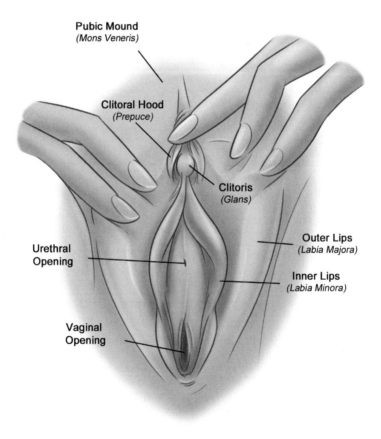

Pubic Mound
(Mons Veneris)

Clitoral Hood
(Prepuce)

Clitoris
(Glans)

Outer Lips
(Labia Majora)

Inner Lips
(Labia Minora)

Urethral
Opening

Vaginal
Opening

may already know that the size, shape and color of labia vary from woman to woman. What you cannot tell from photographs, however, is what's most important: *Sensitivity.*

By design, the outer lips serve to protect the delicate inner workings of the vulva, which fill with blood during arousal, stimulation and pleasure. While your lover undoubtedly enjoys the feelings of gentle touch on her outer lips, be aware this skin is not especially sensitive. For perspective, think how it feels when your lover lightly touches the skin on your scrotum. Sure… that'll awaken you from deep slumber with a pleasant jolt, but you'll probably agree, it's only a fraction of the sensitivity you'll feel as her hands wander north to the tip of your penis.

Just as your sensitivity increases the closer she gets to the head of your penis, your lover's sensitivity takes an arousing leap forward when you venture within her outer lips, too. Think of her inner lips as exquisite delicacies of pleasure—dense with highly sensitive, caress-me-gently nerve endings—where even the gentlest teasing can lift your lover into a pure sexual frenzy. Inner lips were designed by nature to guard your lover's clitoris, but they also crave your touch, which lifts her clitoris out of hiding to greet you as a liberator.

The Clitoris and Clitoral Legs. You've now reached the crown jewel of female sexuality—the epicenter of orgasms—large and seismic, as well as small and exquisite. As you'll find out in Chapter 6, the instant you fine-tune your touch to your lover's clitoral wavelength, you may officially add the title of Sexgod to your name.

The clitoris is densely clustered with so many pleasure-seeking nerve endings, you won't find anything like it anywhere else on her body—or throughout the vast universe. And there's no multi-tasking here! The clitoris is dedicated exclusively to one unique lifetime gig: *Pleasure.*

Interestingly, science has only recently caught up to what history's greatest male lovers somehow always seemed to know: The clitoris you see isn't the clitoris you get—it's merely the tip, also known as the "glans." The full sweep of a woman's pleasure center stems within her pelvis, about two to three inches. It even has a hood, frenulum and shaft that splits into two clitoral legs called "crura," bringing powerful orgasmic delight to every cell in its path. Thank you, dear Mother Nature!

As eye-opening as this discovery is, the main focus of your gentle touch remains the tiny visible portion of the clitoris, so knowing how to find it, and how to caress it, are what separate the boys from the lovers.

How do you find it? You'll find the clitoris atop your lover's two inner lips, cradled just below where they gracefully arc together. Like every snowflake, every clitoris is one-of-a-kind. Some are round, others are oval. Some are prominent, others are hidden. Some are large, others you can barely see. But all that can change during arousal, when the clitoris can grow, and its color can glow, as blood, energy and excitement rush into the area. Remind you of anything?

How do you caress it? The best way to describe the feeling of having it touched is probably close to how the head of your penis feels when your

The Clitoral Legs

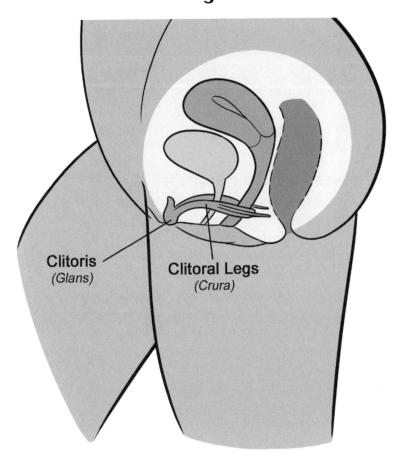

Clitoris
(Glans)

Clitoral Legs
(Crura)

lover touches you. Pretty sexy, huh? What's more, this gives you a giant clue as to what feels good, what leads to orgasm—as well as what leads to yawns and frowns. (More on that later!)

By the way, "clitoris" happens to be the Greek word for "key." Does that mean it's the key to your lover's orgasm? Or the key to you getting more sex? The correct answer is: Why can't it be both?

Clitoral Hood and Commissure. Your lover's clitoris comes with its own tiny hoodie. This soft, fleshy clitoral hood, the "prepuce," is designed to further protect the clitoris—some say it's the female equivalent to a man's fore-skin, which protects the sensitive head of the penis. You can easily glide up the tiny clitoral hood, gently with your fingertip, to reveal your lover's clitoris in all its naked, glistening glory. Was that a gentle moan you heard?

Surrounding the clitoris, like the magnificent setting of a crown jewel, is the "commissure." This, too, feels highly sensitive, and contributes in an erotic way to your lover's arousal and

The Clitoral Hood and Commissure

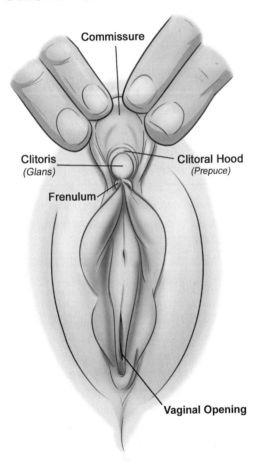

Commissure

Clitoris
(Glans)

Clitoral Hood
(Prepuce)

Frenulum

Vaginal Opening

orgasm. It's what your fingertips and the very tip of your tongue were made for!

The Vagina. Welcome to Intercourse Central— the female's soft, flexible canal designed to embrace your eager, erect penis. Some lucky women are able to achieve purely vaginal orgasms, but most enjoy an assist or a solo from the clitoris. What's surprising to most men is how not-very-sensitive the vagina actually is. Yet what it lacks in sensitivity, it gains in response to pressure and penetration. (Read that last sentence again, because mastering this concept is one more step to being her best lover ever!)

Vulva's Supporting Players

Now that you're familiar with the vulva, here's a quick look at her surrounding pleasures:

Pelvic Floor Muscles. Both women and men have this muscle group underneath the pelvis. It's what contracts rhythmically and involuntarily when you orgasm.

Perineal Sponge. The "G-Spot" is yet another pleasure center for many women. It's located on the upper wall of the vagina, about three-quarters of the way inside. It's not sensitive like a clitoris, but it does respond pleasurably to pressure, and can set off wild orgasms in some women, which can include female ejaculations.

Urethral Opening. The tiny spot where urine flows out of the body. It's located within the vulva, just below the clitoris, and it, too, can be sensitive.

Mons Veneris. The soft, spongy area over the pubic bone. When touched just right, it also plays a role in pleasure.

Perineum. The fleshy, sensitive space between the genitals and the anus where so many women and men love a feeling of gently applied pressure. You may have been calling it by its low-brow name, the "taint."

Anus. The exit that some adults enjoy as an entrance. Yet it can also be highly arousing when lightly touched or slightly penetrated. But that's a subject for another book....

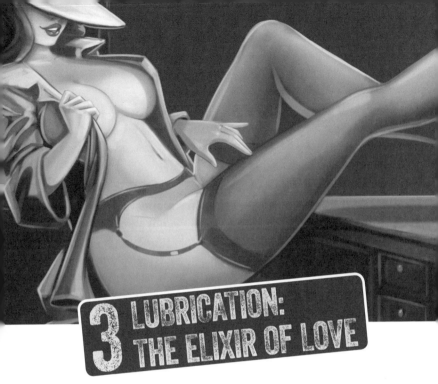

3 LUBRICATION: THE ELIXIR OF LOVE

What if you could double—or even quadruple—the pleasure your lover feels from your every erotic touch? Wouldn't that melt her into your fingers in the slippery-hot frenzy of your wettest dreams?

Or, you can hand her a good case of rug burn, like in her driest nightmares.

The difference can be summed up in one word: Lubrication. And knowing how to start it up—

and keep it up—are your tickets to a joyful slide into Orgasmland.

Stimulated Lubricant

While the vagina is designed to lubricate naturally when aroused, your lover is not a machine. So even after your most valiant efforts, you may still not feel the welcoming signs of enough slipperiness.

Here's why you shouldn't worry: There may be a reason other than the one you're thinking.

Your lover may have taken a medication that dries her out. Stress, breastfeeding, menopause and other hormonal changes can also lead to dryness. Even marijuana can dry out more than one's mouth. And, of course, some women simply produce less lube, no matter how turned on they are.

Fear not! You've got another always-handy, cost-free lube to use as your instant passion-starter: Saliva.

Add saliva to your fingertips and set your glistening fingers free to roam. Once her own vaginal juices start flowing from your slick touch, you're on your way. And remember: Her natural lubrication comes from two tiny ducts to the left and right of her vagina, so roam around to spread it around.

Simulated Lubricant

If you can't keep up with the salivary demand, or your lover prefers longer-lasting, slipperier sensations, you've got plenty of choices that will satisfy both of you immensely. The secret is always to have a good personal lubricant on hand, and within easy reach. Which lubes do you think will put you two over the top?

Water-based Lubricants. This type is the most widely available and your safest, easiest bet. They come in free-flowing liquids, or thicker jellies and gels. You can also choose one that's fruit-flavored to add zest to oral sex.

While a water base provides good slipperiness, these lubes can lose their slick once they get absorbed into the skin. Simply reapply (slather it on!), or use a few drops of water or saliva to bring your lube back to life.

Silicone-based Lubricants. For slip-sliding away and buttplay, silicone rules. It typically lasts longer than water-based lubes, and hardly ever dries out in the heat of passion. Trouble is, it may not offer the best friction for your lover's vulva—and it's more of a challenge for after-sex cleanup. And it seems contrary to common sense, but silicone lubes melt silicone toys. Never use one with the other.

Never-EVER-try Lubes. While nearby kitchen oils, hand lotions or massage oils may seem like a good idea in a pinch, never succumb to temptation with any of these liquids for intimate, off-label use. They are incompatible with healthy sex and can cause unpleasant vaginal infections.

Which Lube for You Two?

Start by asking if your lover has any sensitivities or allergies. Two ingredients you may wish to avoid are glycerin and paraben, which have been removed from many female body-safe elixirs. Heating, flavoring, and tingling ingredients can sometimes cause irritation as well.

If you're new to lube, your best bet is to try a basic water-based formula. These gentle lubes rarely irritate, are odorless, and wash easily out of sheets, bedspreads and auto upholstery. And they're always condom-compatible.

Instant Lube Upgrades

Which sounds better: A drizzle of slippery warm lube on your most sensitive skin, or a sudden splash of arctic-chilled liquid? Next time, try this: Before pouring on the lube, first rub it between your fingers, till the friction heats it up. Even better, place the entire bottle of lube into a bowl of hot water you've thoughtfully placed at bedside. Now you're cookin'!

How much lube is the right amount to squirt? The rule of thumb is, you can never use too much. But if she tells you she's not getting enough friction, you may be over-pouring.

(♥)

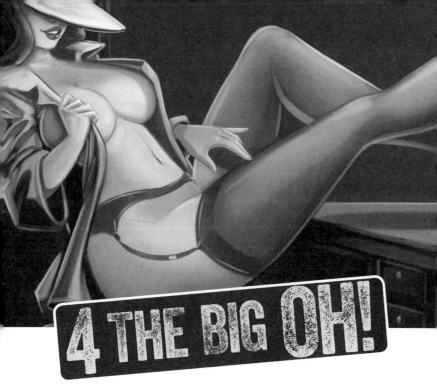

4 THE BIG OH!

Could there possibly be a better-sounding word to capture the pulsating pleasures of sexual release that we humans are so privileged to enjoy?

Orgasm.

These blissful bursts don't just feel extraordinarily good, they're good for us. From their stress-lowering ability to their immune-boosting capability, did you know going without orgasms is actually *un*healthy? Orgasms reset your body systems, help shield you from heart attacks, and even keep your skin looking younger.

If they could bottle it, we'd binge on it.

But there's one rub: Your orgasm is not the same as your lover's orgasm—and if you're treating them as equal, you may be shortchanging her.

As well as yourself.

Tune In to Your Lover's Orgasms

Imagine this: Your lover's warm, slippery fingers joyfully giving you a word-class handjob—but only at the *very bottom* of your penis. How long before you'd go out of your mind?

Just like you (and maybe even more so), your lover needs your sexy touch to land on the right spot—together with a custom tempo, perfect pressure and friction—in order for her to orgasm. In addition, a woman's mind must also be at ease, without worries about kids, deadlines, groceries, or whether she thinks you think she's overweight.

It doesn't require a team of gifted sex researchers to find the ideal spot, tempo and pressure that your lover needs to orgasm. It's entirely your mission, and there's a very easy way to solve this mystery: *Ask!* (In bed, when the moment's right, in the most tender, caring voice you can muster.)

And while you're at it, you can try to set her mind at ease, and focus her entirely on feel-good passion, by summoning up your inner sensitive guy and offering up a few sincere words to help her let go of any worries, and to be with you in the here and now.

Understanding Her Orgasm

What is a female orgasm anyhow? It's the blissful release of sexual tension that takes place during four distinct stages:

1. **Excitement.** This is when foreplay is so very important. It starts the flow of blood to

her erogenous zones: Nipples, clitoris and vulva.

2. **Plateau.** This is when your touch is so meaningful. Her heart starts racing, her breathing quickens, her blood pressure rises, and blood's now rushing to her vulva.

3. **Orgasm.** This is when your sensual clitoral touching is primal. It supercharges the rhythmic, involuntary, oh-so-pleasurable contractions of her pelvic muscles, felt throughout her vulva, uterus, vagina and anus—while her brain sends euphoric chemicals flying!

4. **Resolution.** This is when your understanding of her sudden clitoral oversensitivity is so essential. So her body can relax, and everything can return to normal—perhaps readying for another round.

In the next few chapters, you'll learn many women-endorsed techniques to supercharge clitoral orgasms. But first, it helps to keep a few orgasmic rules-of-thumb in mind:

- A woman usually achieves orgasm between 15 and 40 minutes from the moment you start fooling around, including about 20 minutes of clitoral stimulation. Try to get in sync!

- Less than fifteen percent of women orgasm during intercourse—which means your pre- and during-intercourse clitoral touching takes on added significance.

- Each orgasm has its own personality, depending on the quality of your stimulation, her mood, alcohol consumption, point in her monthly cycle, how she feels about you, how tired she is, how many she's already enjoyed, etc.

- A smallish orgasm can set off three to five bursts of pleasure contractions, while a head-spinning, body-melting orgasm can score as high as 15!

- Some women have yet to learn to orgasm. If your lover tells you she's never climaxed (or only thinks she *may* have), the best solution is for her to try masturbating—while you're not around.

— Some women simply cannot climax, which may be due to emotional issues, medications or menopause. It's not something that you can "fix," but perhaps suggesting a visit to a medical or psychological professional will help.

(♥)

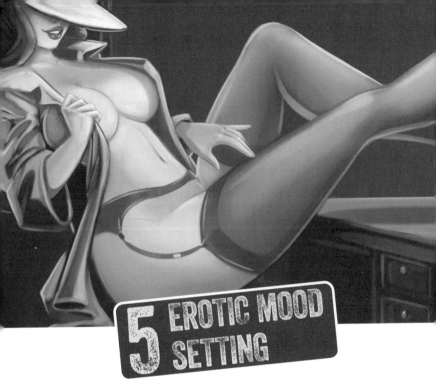

5 EROTIC MOOD SETTING

If you could sit behind a one-way mirror and observe a secret gathering of a dozen sexually active women sipping wine and spilling whines about guys in the sack, what do you supposed you'd hear?

Let's listen in:

"He always pushes too hard and too fast."

"He fancies himself a PORN star."

"He suffers from Eager Dick Syndrome, always trying to stick it in too soon."

"There's no romance anymore."

"He's selfish and grabby in bed."

"He rarely washes his hands, and always needs a shave."

"He thinks my first orgasm's my final orgasm."

"After all these years, he STILL can't touch my clitoris right."

Tough crowd, huh? And that was only the first ten minutes! But here's the good news: If you follow the advice in this book and raise your game even a little, you'll be better than most in bed. And if you raise your game a lot, you'll become a world-class lover.

And the more satisfied your partner is, the more sex she'll want.

Aren't you glad we eavesdropped?

What Does Being "In the Mood" Really Mean?

You're a guy. Which means, in most cases, "ready for sex at any moment." For instance, at *this* moment. Right?

Conversely, most women will rarely drop their panties at the drop of a hat. And *there's* the disconnect. So to get in sexual sync, she either needs to speed up, or you need to slow down— and we know who'll win that contest of wills (especially if you want good sex, or even any sex at all!).

There are several reasons why women take longer to warm up. And if you take a moment to understand them, and accommodate them, you'll discover the true seductive magic of a woman's erotic awakening—if you can somehow keep your autopilot fly from unzipping itself!

Physically, a woman needs more of the right kind of stimulation to increase blood flow to her erogenous zones. During this pulse-quickening blood-rush, her erectile tissue and sex receptors grow excited, sparking a sexual frenzy that feels so good to her, it feeds the drive to explore your body with equal gusto.

On the other hand, what do you think happens when you pounce too fast? You short-circuit a natural progression in her that's evolved over thousands of years, and can easily be summed up in one self-evident word:

"OUCH!"

Is that the sound you want to hear? Or would your rather hear a breathless *"Ohhhwwwhhh"* as she seductively unzips you herself, while you thank your lucky stars you were wise enough to take your fly off autopilot.

So Far, So Good. Here's Where Others Blow It.

You're both piping hot. Clothes are flying through the air. And your penis keeps throbbing uncontrollably. Now's the time to dive in for the ol' plunge 'n pump, right?

Hey…are you on the clock? Settle down. YOU may be piping hot, but she may not be piping anything. And at this rate, you'll never solve "The Mystery of the Undercover Clitoris" if you keep ignoring her crown jewel altogether.

The sly little secret? Move slowly, move gently, and tease her to come to you.

The fast, crazy action you crave will come later, when your skills have lifted her up to your frenzied level of passion. And it won't take long, if you follow this advice:

Start with light stroking over her entire body. Gently massage her inner thighs. Squeeze her butt. Slowly scratch her mound with your nails. Tease her vulva with your fingertips. Drizzle in a little lube. Do you feel her starting to gyrate towards you, and not away? That's the sign you're looking for, because it means you're awakening the erectile tissue in her vulva—especially in her clitoris—and she wants more.

So give her more!

Tease the entrance to her vagina with your loving fingertips, but don't slip inside. Now gently glide your fingertips toward the top of her vulva, like you're about to touch her clitoris, *but don't!* Instead, slide gently around it, till her body begs you to touch it. That's when you know she's ready to have it touched. So touch it, but only for a moment—then slide your fingertip all around the rest of her vulva.

Let her clitoris chase your fingertip!

Ready to take her passion to an even higher level? With your full palm lightly pressing onto her mound, send your fingertips sliding down the sides of her inner lips, merely side-swiping her clitoris. Your gentle pressure will excite all her pleasure producing nerve endings, including her clitoral legs under the surface!

What If Her Clitoris Is SUPER-Sensitive?

Does too much of a good thing exist in sex? For some women, yes. The clitoris is so sensitive, direct contact can actually hurt.

Your lover will surely yelp if super sensitivity causes her discomfort, and here's what you do with this information: Believe her, no matter what experiences you've had with other women.

In all likelihood, your lover will still be able to enjoy a clitoral orgasm, but only from indirect contact all around it. *Please don't make her have to remind you not to touch it directly (and heed any other directions she gives), because her irritation will only grow.* Your mission is to find what she DOES like, and repeat it as often as you can.

What If Your Moves Still Aren't Working?

Sometimes, even the most skilled lovers with the hottest hands don't register more than an "eh." Not to worry, all is not lost. Keep these potential sexbusters in mind:

- ➤ How cold is the room? If she's chilly, flip on the heat—or turn off the A/C.

- ➤ Have you bypassed the long, passionate kissing she loves? Get sensual.

- ➤ Are you rubbing her too hard? Soft 'n gentle is the key.

- Are you rubbing her too fast? Take it slow, then ask if she wants faster.

- Is the lube drying out? Then pour on more. Nothing dampens a woman's mood more than an annoying touch of a dry finger.

- Is her head just not in the game? Take a breather, and refocus her attention on your affection.

- Is your environment romantic? Ask her what music she'd like to hear, or dim the lights way down low.

- If you forgot to shower and shave, be sure to remember for next time. Clean and smooth is sexy.

- Show up with clean, trimmed, filed fingernails. She'll appreciate that.

- Or simply ask: "Do you like when I do this?" or "Would you like it softer?" Your proactive asking will help open healthy lines of communication.

(♥)

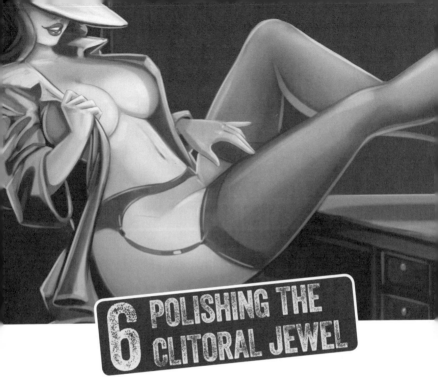

6 POLISHING THE CLITORAL JEWEL

"If men ever figure out how to please the clitoris, we might actually achieve world peace."

— ANONYMOUS

Of course, who knows how this could speed up global warming?

But this is really about you, not mankind. And it all comes down to pleasing your woman in the sack, so she'll truly see you as her Lover with a capital L.

Sound good? Then please do this: Read the rest of this book at a slow, easy pace. Feel your inspiration (and libido) rise, absorb all these insights, and plan your moves till they're firmly in your bone, *er*...bones!

Ready? Let's get started....

Master Class #1: Hearing Is Not Listening

You hear what's going on around you, of course, but when you truly listen, you pick up additional, often subtle clues about what all those sounds really mean. Experienced lovers not only listen with their ears—they use all their senses to know whether their partner is deep in ecstasy, or drowsy in apathy.

From now on, tune in to your lover. Listen to her body. Hear her sounds. Feel her warmth. Breathe her scent. See her glisten. Sense her passion. If the signals you're picking up are stimulating and provocative, congratulations! Keep doing what you're doing. If the signals are mixed, or missing, change course till you find what works.

Master Class #2: Mystery Loves Company

Maybe you're a guy who'll keep driving all night instead of asking directions, but bring that philosophy into the bedroom, and you'll likely be driving alone.

Nine out of ten women will be overjoyed if you crack the ice by simply asking what they like, as long as you're passionate, respectful and patient. (And by the way, that tenth woman isn't worth your time!)

In fact, your lover's response to a softly spoken question or two can be the difference between fumbling in the dark or falling into ecstasy. It's rarely awkward or embarrassing, if you simply slip in your question organically...like this:

"A little slower?"

"This feel good?"

"Softer...?"

"Better...?"

"Up here…?"

"Little more lube?"

You get the picture. Simple, easy, sincere. No multiple choices. No essays. And then, don't be surprised if your lover's answers don't come in words, but in sensual *Mmmmmms* or *Aaaaah-hhhs*. That's fine, because it's all you need. And squirming away from you, or an *"OW!!"* are certainly self-explanatory. But the key to all this is to *respond* to her feedback by giving her what she craves. And when you ultimately deliver what she's guiding you towards, passion zooms like a rocket!

Master Class #3: Micro-touching for Miracles

On the previous pages, you observed how to find the clitoris. In later pages, you're going to see the wildest touches and positions you could ever try. And here, you're going to see how subtle micro-touches can turn even the most shy, reserved, librarian-type woman into your passion-charged lover.

Go light 'n slow. Most women prefer a lover with a slow hand, at least until they're in overdrive. You'll find that your slow, gentle touch will arouse your lover better and faster than a hard and fast touch, no matter what you think you've learned in well-acted pornos. How do you know the right soft touch? Easy: Start with the same soft pressure you'd use to brush your fingertips across your eyelashes, and adjust from there.

Pause. Want to blast your lover into orbit? Do the opposite of what you'd expect, and try holding perfectly still. That's right. The next time she's riding a wave of fingertip ecstasy, hold your hand steady, and see what happens. You may find she starts pressing and rubbing her hot, moist vulva onto you!

Surround. Instead of pouncing on her clitoris like a cat on a mouse, try encircling her jewel with small rings of pleasure, using only your gentle, moist fingerpad. Often, indirect pleasure is all she craves, at least until she's warmed up, on the verge of coming, or even the entire time. It's up to you to find out.

Vary it. You're not a robot, so don't pleasure her like one. Instead of touching her the same way all the time, vary your stroking pace and techniques to create even more pleasure. Just remember: When she says breathlessly, "Just like THAT"—then *that's* exactly what you continue doing, because you've just struck gold!

Surface area. Instead of a fingertip, try touching with the sensual flat part of your fingers—the finger*pads.* This exquisite sensation is loved by most women, especially at first touch. As lubrication increases, try spreading the slipperiness around with all four of your fingerpads, slowly, gently, up and down her vulva. Depending on your position, you can also excite her with your lubed *thumbpad.* This gives her an ideal surface to grind her red-hot clitoris on.

Lube it. You know how different a dry handjob feels from a wet slippery handjob. Now triple that difference—and you can guess how unlubricated touching feels on your lover's vulva. (Some women say it feels like sandpaper!) Just add a few drops of saliva or some good lube, and turn irritation into exhilaration.

Be ambidextrous. Clitoral touching isn't just for fingertips. Wiggle your tongue, wag your penis, nudge your nose, bring in a sex toy (or two!). And don't forget what you just read directly above!

Flattery. Every woman appreciates a sincere compliment. Hairstyle, clothing, scent. But have you ever remarked how beautiful she looks down there? While you're exploring, find a position so you can see what you're doing. Then offer up your compliments. Just be aware: A completely sincere expression of, "You have a beautiful pussy," will flatter one woman, but send another running for her coat. (If there's any doubt, simply say, "beautiful flower" or just "beautiful.")

Master Class #4: Romancing the Clitoris

If you've followed this advice, and all is going well, your lover will reach the plateau stage—that wonderful space between mild touch and wild orgasm. Now's your chance to show her what a good lover you really are.

First, if vulva and fingers aren't super slippery

already, add some lube and spread it all around. Now place her clitoris between your thumb and index finger, and with ever-so-gentle pressure, let it slip around. If she responds well, try adding a little extra pressure. Or back off if you sense it's too much.

When her clitoris becomes erect, try touching it over and across, and in small circles. If she likes that, go a little faster. If you sense you're going too fast, hold still for a moment to let her overstimulation subside, then resume when she's ready. Now you know her max pleasure speed, too!

If your partner loves direct clitoral stimulation, try tapping her clitoris, ever so gently. Vary your speed and pressure. Try four or five taps in a row, then pause till she begs for more, or reaches up to tap back at your finger with her clitoris!

Becoming a master of clitoral stimulation puts you in a top tier of lovers, because too few guys ever figure this out. Too bad! Your lover totally craves it, and here's why: When she feels your gentle caress, her slippery clitoris and all the

$\left(\heartsuit\right)$

surrounding area will grow fully aroused, as her entire body quivers with delight. And that's the passion that comes back to you many times over.

Master Class #5: Read Her Lips

Unlike your lover's ultra-sensitive clitoris, her labia may crave direct stimulation, and not the ever-so-gentle clitoral-type touch either. Here, touching too gently can actually feel a bit boring.

A woman's outer lips love to be touched, squeezed and massaged. How do you know if your touch is too much? Simply use the same comfortable pressure you'd use on your own earlobes. Then it's simply a matter of following your lover's lead: The more excited she gets, the more stimulation you give.

Your lover's inner lips, however, may desire a gentler, more teasing touch. Find her wavelength, and you might bring her to orgasm with your labial artistry alone—which she will reward you for many times over, especially if direct clitoral touch is too over-stimulating for her.

Master Class #6: The Entire Vulva and Beyond

Some guys are labia lovers, some are clitoral connoisseurs, but the best lovers know how to please every nook and cranny within a woman's entire vulva. The vulva is one sexy erogenous playground, all interconnected, with plenty of erotically different sensations to enjoy.

Try running your lubed fingertip from the very top, above the clitoral hood, down and throughout all the fleshy crevices along the way. Massage all four lips simultaneously. Use the side of your hand, or the flat of your palm, not just your fingertips. Spread all the lube around. Even the most prim and proper lady will let go of daintiness in favor of sloppy and messy in the heat of passion.

Now, for extra credit, reach up with your free hand and play with her breasts. Then use your mouth for kissing and nibbling her body.

Master Class #7: Orgasmic Tipping Pointers

What do you do when she's on the verge of orgasm—that sweet spot between maximum sexual tension and full-on pulsating release? Here's what you *don't* do: Lose focus.

Stay with her, picking up your pace at just the right tempo for her erotic contortions and exotic moans. Resist sprinting for the finish line. Instead, do something unexpected: Pause, just as her body needs your touch the most. As she goes wild, restart slowly, teasing her beyond any pleasure she's ever felt.

When she's close to going over the edge, pick up your pace a little, and keep your rhythm steady. Let *her* find the tipping point. If you try to force it, or go too fast, you'll probably lose her. Stay with her, and you'll truly be her Jedi Sexknight.

(♥)

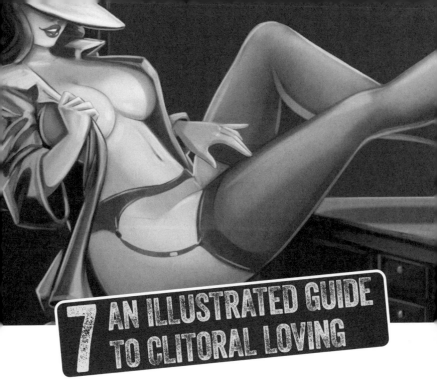

7 AN ILLUSTRATED GUIDE TO CLITORAL LOVING

If a picture is worth a thousand words, how many words do the stunning illustrations in this chapter put in *your* head?

These touching techniques are guaranteed to bring your lover pure sexual ecstasy—while you get full credit, along with her undying passion-in-return. (Note: Guarantee is null and void if you neglect to lube properly!)

Lube up and have fun!

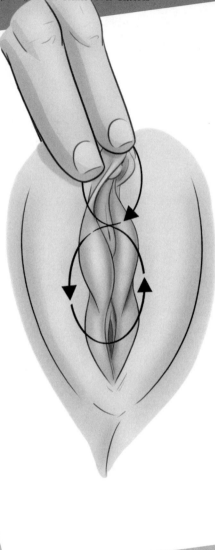

8th Wonder of the World

Ever so lightly, run a fingerpad (or two) up and down your lover's vulva, in a classic "figure 8" pattern. Gradually increase pressure, and see whether she loves when you merely graze her clitoris, or caress it directly. For extra thrills, stroke from one through ten with your fingertips—or spell out her name!

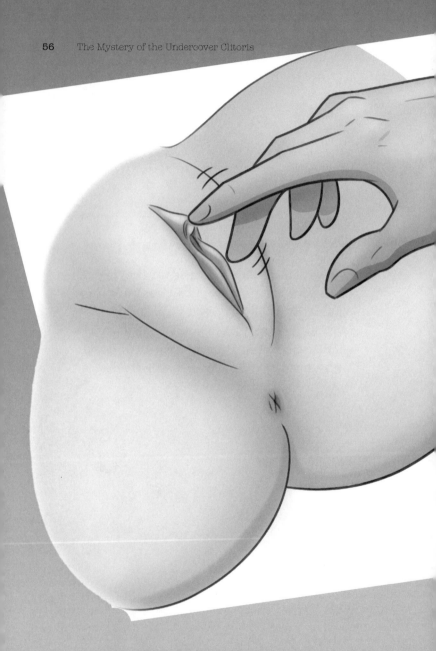

Walk of Fame

Make like your two fingers are "walking," and stroke your lover's inner vulva, slowly at first, then with a little more speed and pressure. Travel up and down the length of the vulva, and tease the clitoris a little each time you're there. Don't be robotic—vary the pace and pressure till you find what rocks her world.

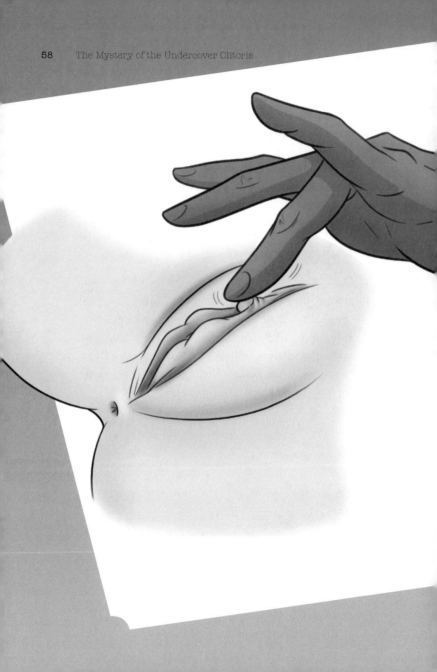

Touch 'n Go

Ever so lightly, tease her clitoris with your fingerpad (don't treat it like a doorbell, or you'll be shown the door!). See if your lover prefers very light stimulation on only the tip of her clitoris, or enjoys a little more pressure. Or try this: Touch everywhere *around* her clitoris, but never directly on it.

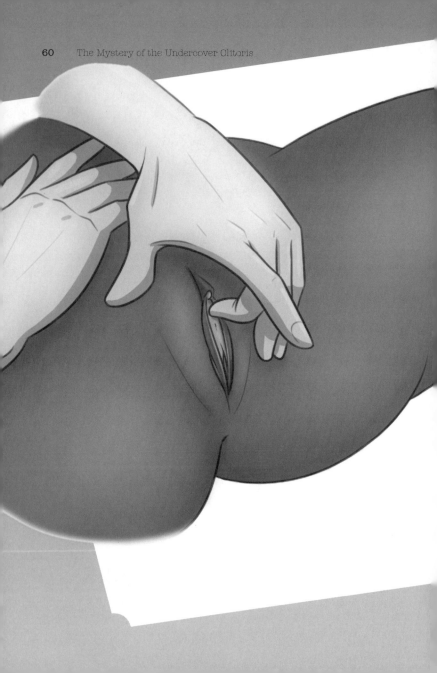

Slow Tease

Teasing can drive your lover insane—in a good way! Try this: Starting at the mouth of her vagina, s-l-o-w-l-y stroke up the middle using your fingerpad till you reach her clitoris, then return to her vagina and repeat. Continue the slow tease till she begs you to touch her clitoris.

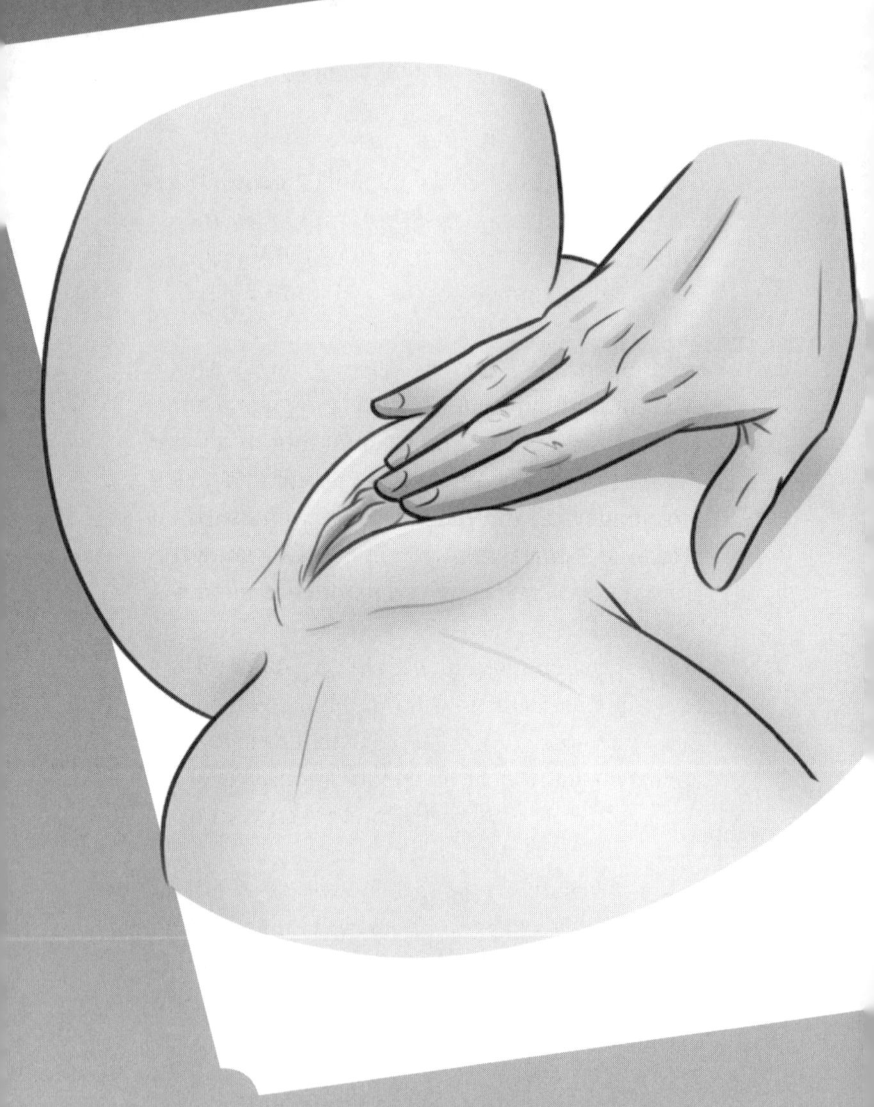

Press to Play

Using the broad, flat part of your hand and several fingers side-by-side, press lightly onto your lover's entire vulva, treating her to full labia and clitoral contact, along with lots of lube. Vary your massaging style, rhythm and pressure till her hips move gleefully with your touch.

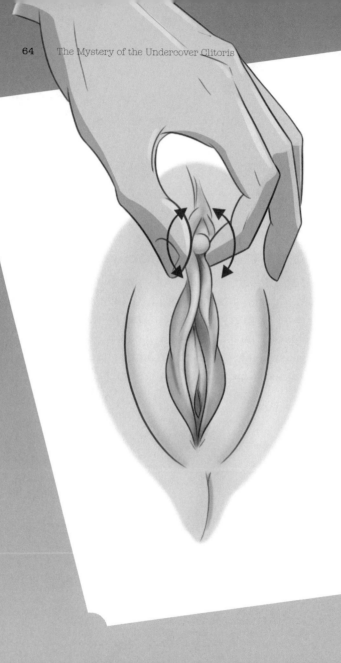

Orgasmic Twirl

This will surely feel big to your lover, but it's a tiny masterpiece for you. Once you locate her pre-heated erect clitoris, surround it with your thumb and forefinger, and squeeze it ever so delicately. Now, try a soft, slow roll, followed by delicate stroking up and down her labia. Please don't attempt this without lube!

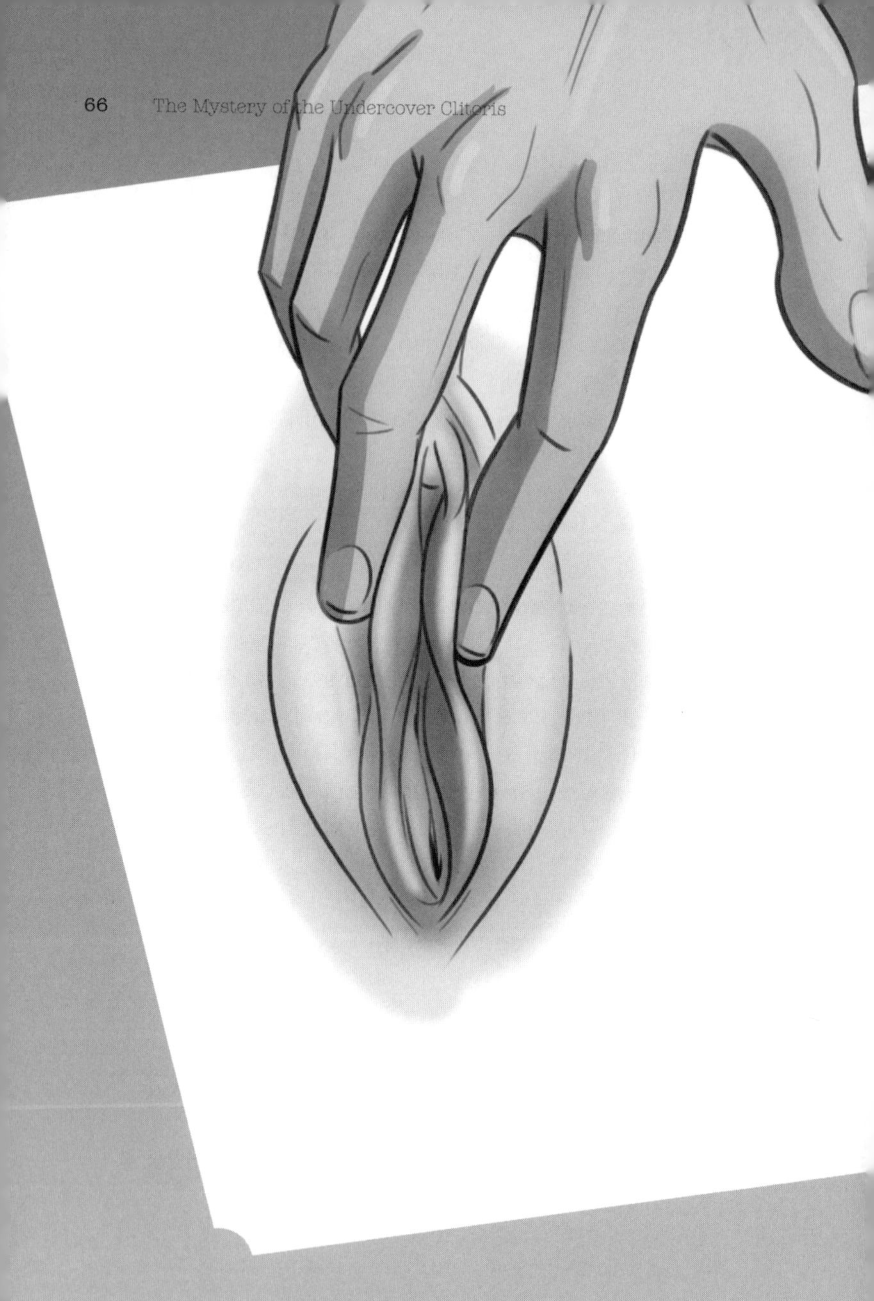

Velvet Sideswipe

Slide the sides of your lubed fingertips slowly down her inner labia and back up again, using only light pressure. All that pleasurable moving and pushing around her labia will indirectly heat up her clitoris and clitoral legs under the surface. Some women find this even better than direct clitoral touching. What about *your* lover?

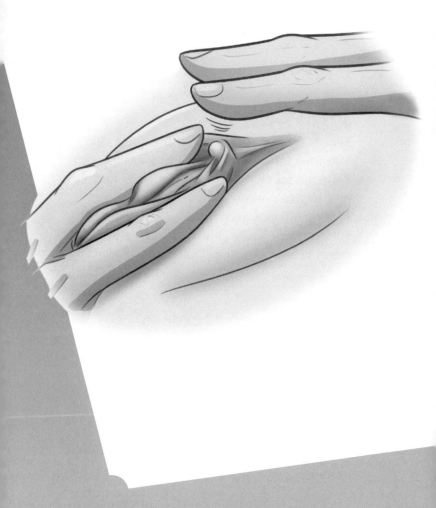

What's on Tap?

Clitoral tapping isn't for every woman, but if your lover is one of the lucky few, this move will ignite her soul. With one of your hands, gently separate her labia. With your other hand, lightly tap with your fingerpad (or three!). If she grows more aroused, increase your speed slowly. You can even take it from tap to slap, as long as it's light and gentle.

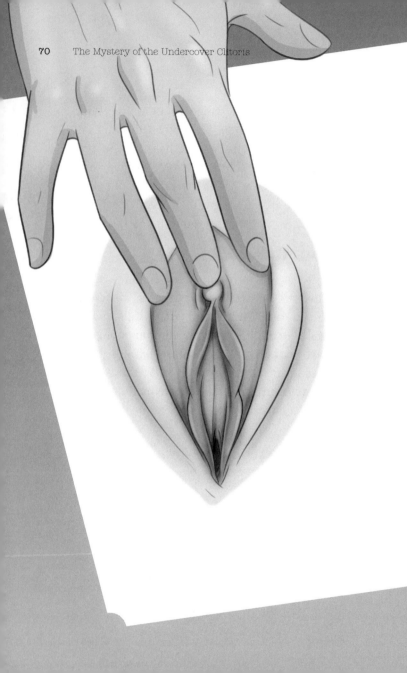

Three's Company

Spread open your lover's labia with your index and ring fingers. Now your middle finger is in perfect position to stimulate her fully revealed clitoris. This works best if your lover is a fan of direct clitoral contact. Now move all three fingers down to the mouth of her vagina, then back up again. What are you doing now with your *free* hand?

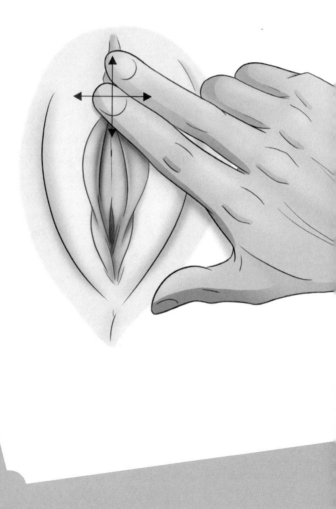

Erotic Fingerpainting

Think of yourself as the world's foremost erotic fingerpainter, in the midst of creating a sensual masterpiece. And while you're at it, you'll also discover your lover's most sensitive, arousable spots. Experiment with pace and pressure, and don't limit yourself to right angles, Picasso!

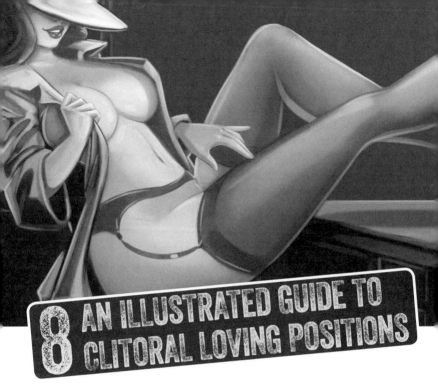

8 AN ILLUSTRATED GUIDE TO CLITORAL LOVING POSITIONS

There's a sexual screwball flying your way, spun by a pitching ace named Mother Nature. And if you don't get wood on it, you'll find yourself warming the bench while everyone else scores.

Better yet, you can master it—and triumph with walk-off home runs. Every time.

What's so screwy? You'll surely agree how magnificently your erect penis aligns with your lover's excited vagina. But what if your loving partner doesn't see it exactly the same way? What if, thanks to an odd quirk of biology, the one very special matchup she loves and craves is too often left out of the mix?

That matchup is direct clitoral stimulation— the glorious contact most every woman needs to orgasm. In fact, multiple sex surveys show that 80 to 90 percent of women do *not* orgasm during vaginal intercourse—mainly because the female orgasm trigger is getting little or no direct stimulation.

Relax! It's not your fault. But since we can't change this quirk of biology, it's up to you to change. And by simply including the erotic clitoral contact you'll see demonstrated in this chapter, you'll be able to skyrocket her orgasms in quantity *and* duration *and* strength. And you'll likely fulfill her desire to climax during intercourse—even simultaneously with you!

And that's a genuine walk-off Grand Slam! Each and every time.

How to Add In What Nature Left Out

Be open. Give yourself time and patience to become familiar with the motions and positions she craves. Here's how: *Ask. Listen. Act.* You may discover she's in a bucking crazy mood one moment, and in a highly clitoral no-penetration mood the next. That's your hint on how to be her ideal lover, at every given moment. Take that hint.

Slow down. Do you suffer from EDS? That's Eager Dick Syndrome, and there's no magic pill to cure it. You simply need to slow yourself down, and tease her with your magic fingertips, till she's warmed up and ready for you to bring your penis to the party.

Get creative. Take your stimulation techniques off auto-pilot and vary your clitoral touching till you find what she likes. Instead of one fingertip, try two or three, or your outstretched palm, or your fleshy thumbpad, or the tip of your penis, or even your nose! As long as your lover likes it, you will, too.

Master the Secrets of Star-Quality Sex

Get slippery! No matter what you've watched on the Internet, no woman is ready for intercourse unless she's fully lubricated. Rather than pushing into dryness, you have three good choices: You can continue exciting her with foreplay to stimulate her natural lubrication. You can drizzle on some of the slippery sex lube you've wisely purchased in advance. Or best yet, you can touch her to glorious first orgasm with what you've learned in this book. She'll then be totally lubricated AND sporting the biggest smile you've ever seen.

Thrust not. Vigorous pornstar pumping should only be ONE of your gears—and saved for the right time. Instead, try some slow rocking, or grinding, or even perfect stillness while inside. Pressing your fleshy pubic mound into her clitoris ever so lovingly could set off the spark that leads to the mutual thrusting you love.

Go selfie! If your fingers don't quite reach from the position you're in, and she's craving direct clitoral stimulation, you still have another good option: Encourage her to touch herself. If she's the shy type, try gently guiding her hand to let her know it's okay—and she may simply take over from there.

Check in. I can't say this often enough. If you don't know what she's craving in the moment, then ask. She may reveal your moves are too subtle, or too rough. And that's okay, because her honest guidance will help you fine-tune your touch to the tempo she's craving. And that's when primal passion takes over.

Lastly, it's all too easy to get lost in your own good feelings. After all, there's nothing more exhilarating than that warm wet tightness of being inside. But if you truly wish to be a world-class lover, you can't get so distracted that you forget you're not alone.

Try slowing it down, tuning into her needs and desires, and being a generous lover.

Your rewards will come. Again and again.

And again.

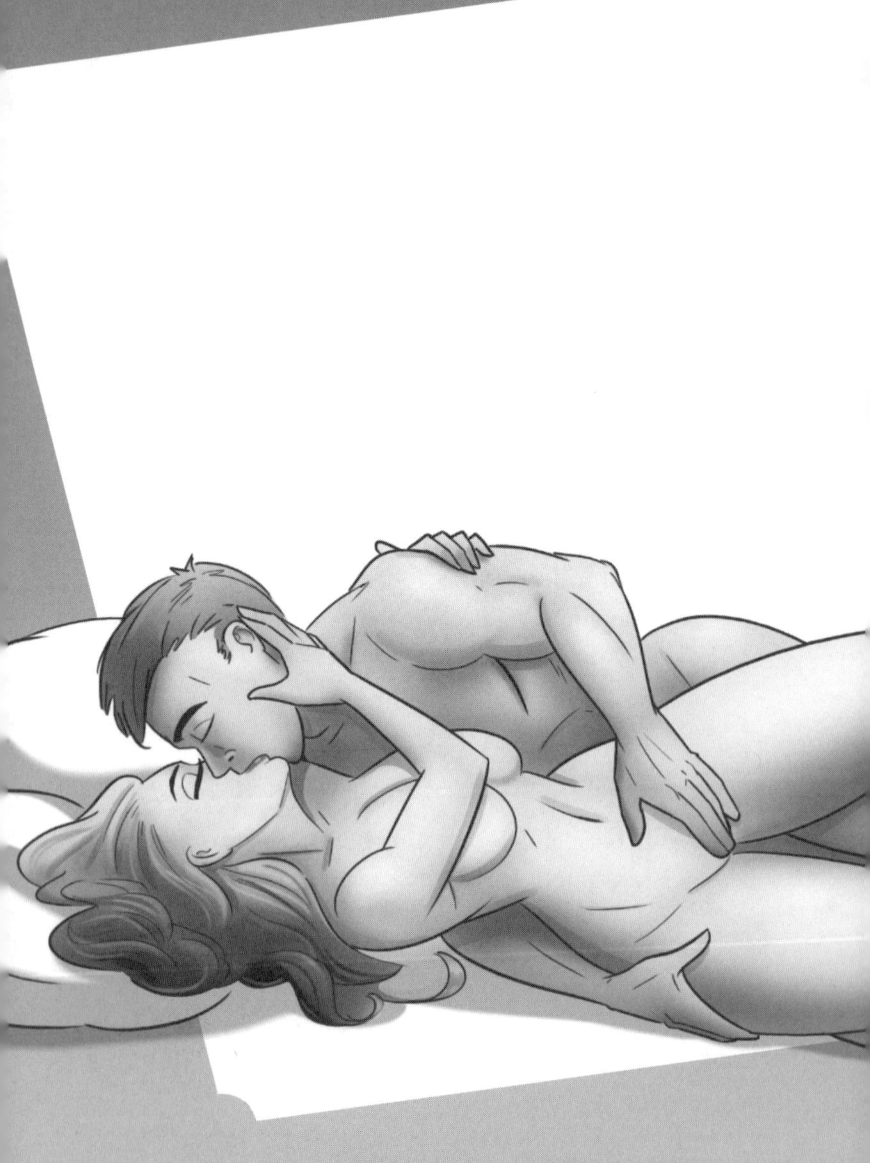

Tangled Up in You

With all the sensual skin-on-skin contact, "spooning" is truly a deep lovemaking experience—and a favorite position of many women. It also gives your hands freedom to touch her with newfound passion. But instead of going in right away, start with seductive teasing. Slowly glide your fingertips near her yearning clitoris, tempting her with Chapter 7's "Velvet Sideswipe" (p.67). When she's moaning with excitement and craving more, move to the "8th Wonder of the World" (p.55) and spell out, *I love you* with gentle fingertip motion.

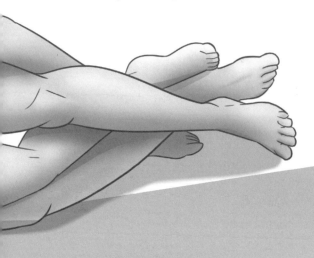

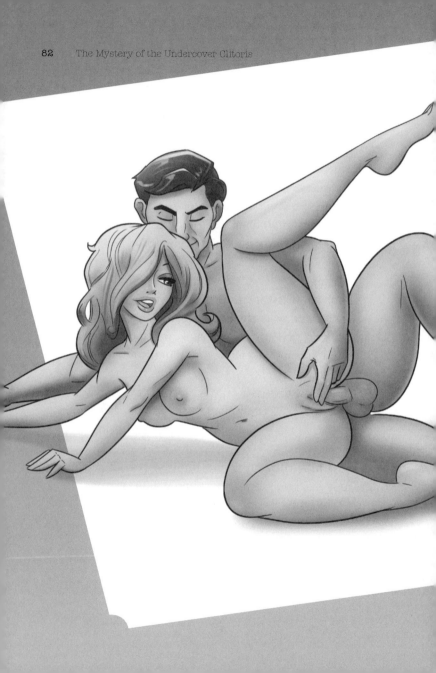

All Access Pass

Spooning's fun and intimate, but when passions heat to a frenzy, you may find your bodies revving beyond that position's slower pace. "All Access Pass" is an easy upgrade that gives you more freedom to move, while maintaining that delicious skin-on-skin contact. Try "Press to Play" (p. 63) or "Orgasmic Twirl" (p. 65) as you whisper sexy thoughts in her ear.

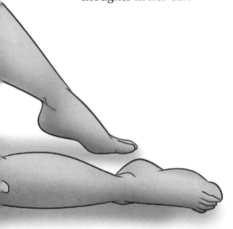

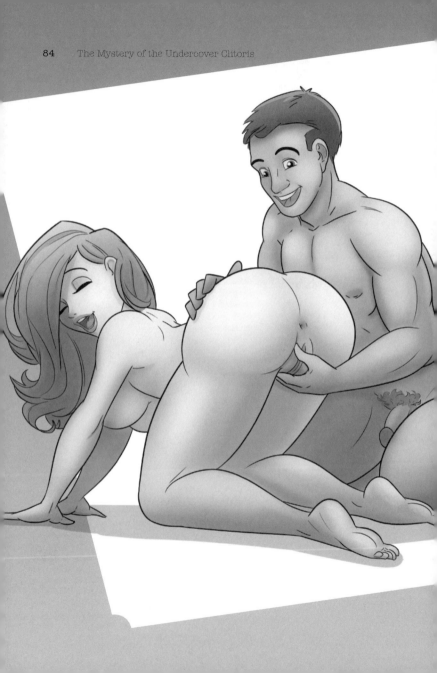

Moon Goddess

This erotic "doggy-style" clitoral stimulating position is the perfect preamble to come-from-behind lovemaking. Position yourself for the best comfort and angle, and take your time finding the tempting touches that'll drive her insane. When she's fully aroused and yearning for the next level, move into lovemaking—but don't stop the clitoral stroking! You'll find this is one of the easiest and most comfortable positions for you to touch her clitoris while you're inside her. And since you're a world-class lover, what do you plan to do with your free hand?

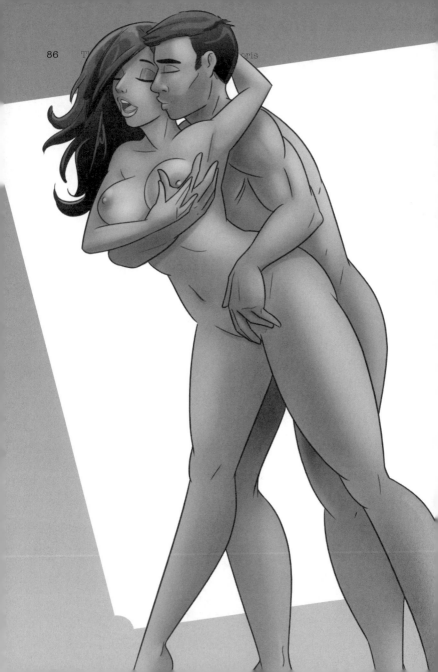

Come from Behind

Earn a standing ovation tonight! While you're behind her, glide your fingertips all over her body, then slowly inch them toward her vulva. This is the perfect time to seduce her with your soft kisses and gentle neck nibbles. You can even place one of her feet on a sturdy chair, exposing her flower for even more of your orgasmic touch. She'll enjoy any of the erotic touching techniques, but only a true master can handle the "Slow Tease" (p. 61) for more than a few seconds!

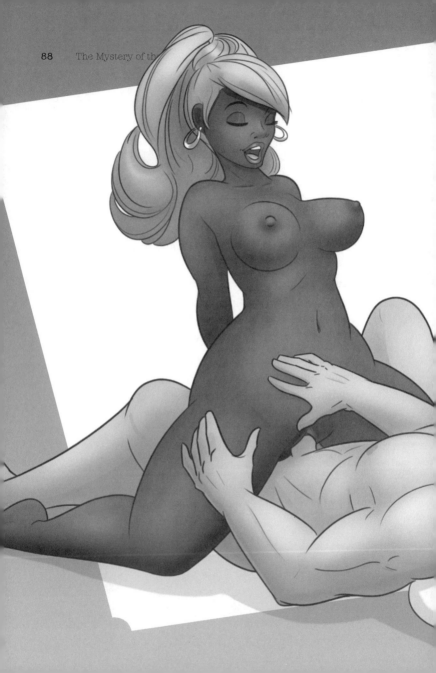

Thumb Like It Hot

Can you guess why this is a doubly orgasmic position for her? Not only is she in charge of her own grinding and thrusting, but with some gentle thumb play from you, she'll soon take off like a rocket. Best yet, try holding still. That's right! Let *her* make love to *you,* stroking against your still thumbpad and grinding on your stiff penis and pubic mound at the exact tempo and pressure she desires. Then all you have to do is watch the pleasure show unfolding right before your eyes!

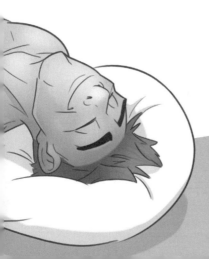

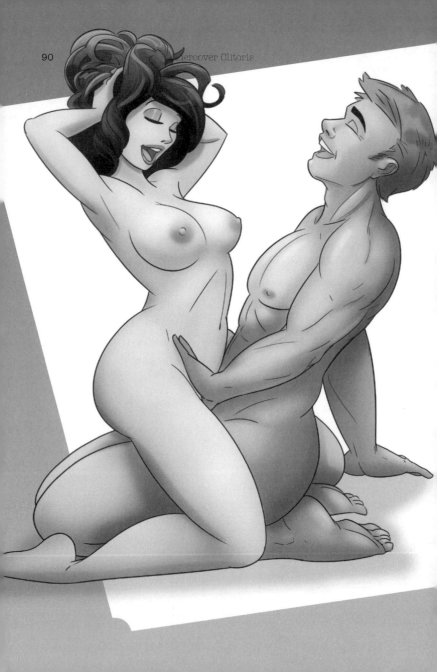

Bucking Cowgirl

This fun variation on the "cowgirl" position allows you to pleasure her clitoris easily with your golden thumbpad. Or, she may prefer to take full control of the gyrating and pressure on her clitoris against your thumbpad—so stay in tune with her. Then try wrapping your free arm around her hips and hold her tight—this will add support for her grinding and thrusting. Does she enjoy when you caress and kiss her or gaze deeply into her eyes? Can you think of a better time?

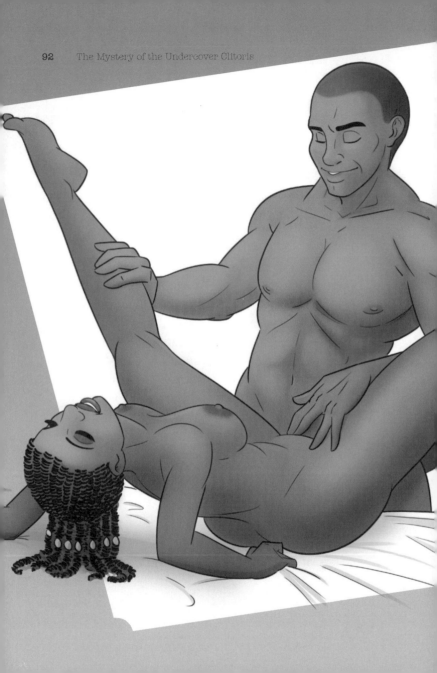

Wish Maker

This edge-of-your-seat (or bed!) position maximizes your control of thrusting and gives each of you plenty of eye candy, too. Slowly tease her vulva with the "Walk of Fame" (p. 57) or "Erotic Fingerpainting" (p. 73) touching techniques, then switch it up to some focused thumbpad action, rubbing in circles around her clitoris. When she's really warmed up, see how she likes even more contact, and rub her with the lubricated base of your palm. What's next? Why not invite her fingers to the party—and enjoy all the eye candy you can devour!

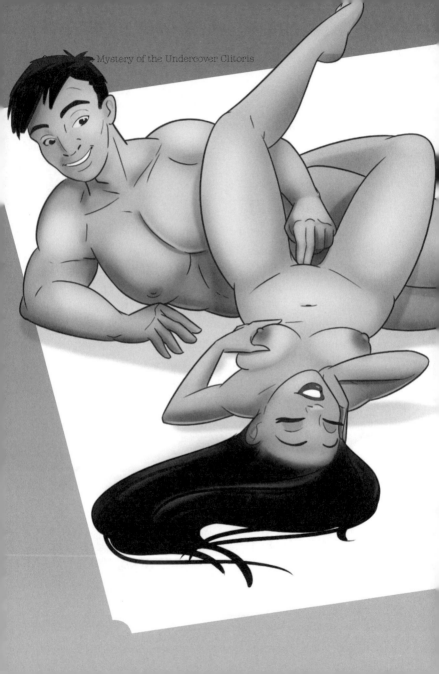

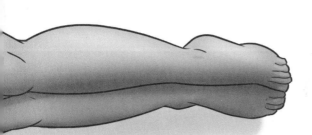

Touch for Joy

If you've been feeling a little in the dark about touching her vulva, this exciting position lets you view exactly how each of your sensual touches arouse her. Try pleasing her with your fingertips, or explore thumbpad caresses while you're inside. Remember, she may prefer you to hold still so she can do the grinding at her own pace and pressure, while enjoying your clitoral touching. And since she has both hands free to roam all over her body, she can enhance your touch with wild improvised stimulations of her own.

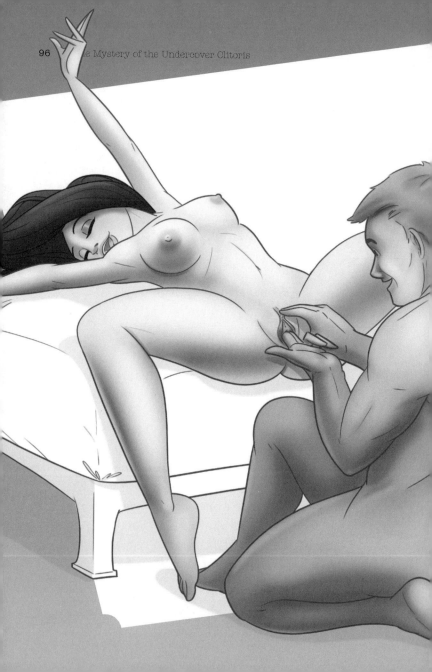

Pussycat's Meow

With all four hands free to roam, each of you can easily enhance the touch of the other. While you gently penetrate her with the fingers of one hand, your other hand is free to caress her clitoris into an orgasmic frenzy. And she's free to raise the heat with self-pleasure, or just sprawl out and let you work your own erotic magic. What a view!

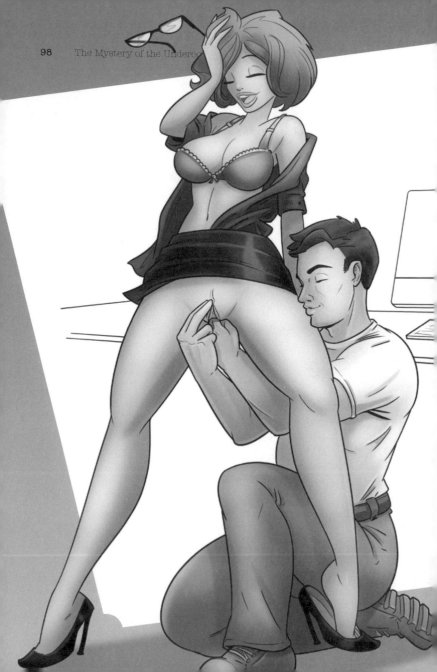

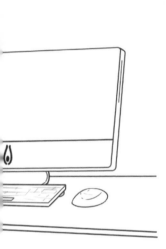

Better Than a Coffee Break

This kneeling-style pleasure position comfort-ably and naturally curves your wrists and fingers to play her vulva with the creativity of a concert pianist. And remember: Your fingers bend in ways that your penis can't, so why not curl them slightly while inside and caress her G-Spot, or wiggle and vibrate them at a sensual pace that lifts her feet off the ground?

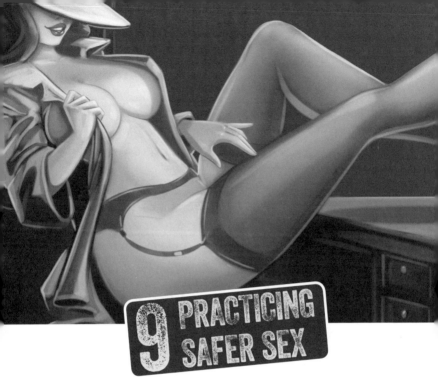

9 PRACTICING SAFER SEX

With sex comes risk. No human being on earth is immune to today's menu of sexually transmitted infections (STIs)—including you. You *must* protect yourself.

To practice safer sex means to keep the bodily fluids that can transmit STIs totally separate (blood, semen and vaginal secretions). Being prepared shows that you are considerate to your partner and that you care about yourself.

The good news? Safer sex doesn't have to slow you down. In fact, you'll find it actually enhances the mood, since you'll both spend far less time worrying—and far more time loving.

So put your most powerful sex organ to work for you: Your brain. Practice the safety precautions in this chapter. Your health—and life—depend on it.

Safer Sex—Here's How

There's only one way to decrease your chances of contracting or transmitting STIs: Practice safer sex—each and every time.

You're mostly safe kissing, licking, nibbling, sucking and massaging your lover everywhere but on the genitals (but you can catch cold sores if your partner has them on the mouth). And you're mostly safe bringing your lover to orgasm with the clitoral fingertip-touching techniques in this book—as long as you keep your partner's body fluids from entering your body, either through an orifice or a cut in your skin.

Here are the practical steps you can take:

Use latex condoms. Without fail, roll a fresh latex condom over the penis before it ever touches the vagina, mouth or anus. Roll them over sex toys, too. Always use sex lubes that are "latex-compatible," such as water-based varieties. And store condoms away from heat.

Use latex barriers. For penetrative fingerplay, wear a latex glove or a "finger cot"—a snug latex cover that rolls onto your finger.

Use lubricant. It not only makes it more comfortable for her—it also helps prevent any tearing of latex condoms.

Stay sober. Alcohol and recreational drugs weaken your resolve. Know when to say "when."

Wash up. Before anyone touches anything, wash hands with antibacterial soap and warm water. And file nails smooth.

Be a neat lover. Toss all used condoms in the trash, and throw after-sex towels into the hamper.

Answer Key

How'd you do?

1. Where do you find the clitoris?
   a) Halfway inside the vagina
   b) Atop the inner folds of the vulva
   c) At the tip of the uvula
Turn to Chapter 2 for a life-sized view!

2. About how big is an average clitoris?
   a) The size of a small pea
   b) The size of a little toe
   c) The size of an un-erect penis
Really! See Chapter 2 for an inside view!

3. What's the correct pronunciation of "clitoris?"
   a) Kli-TOR-us
   b) KLIT-a-ris
   c) Kli-tor-US
Both a and b are considered to be correct.

4. What's the best way to touch a clitoris?
   a) Hard and fast
   b) Soft and gentle
   c) Around it, indirectly
It depends on what your lover likes, how aroused she is, and how close she is to climaxing. See Chapter 6.

(♥)

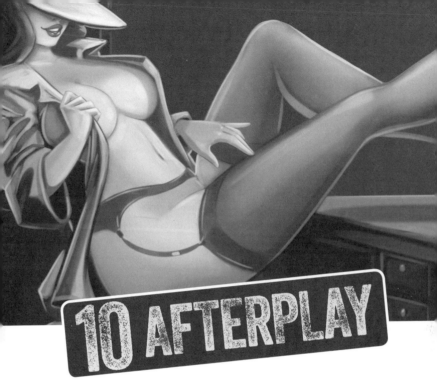

10 AFTERPLAY

Inspired? Eager? Horny? All of the above?

Now that you're fully empowered, imagine how your lover will feel the moment you spring your newfound talents on her. It could be the beginning of an endless, upward spiral of passion, rewarding you in ways you can't imagine.

Be a generous lover. This means thinking of your partner's pleasure before your own. After all, when both of you are generous, the passion comes back to each of you, surging stronger with each lusty touch.

And be patient! This isn't a race. Live in the moment. Discover the joys of touching in slow motion, until passions naturally speed things into the heated sexual frenzy you came for. Your lover will be eternally grateful.

You want to become a Jedi Sexknight? *This is how.*

(♥)

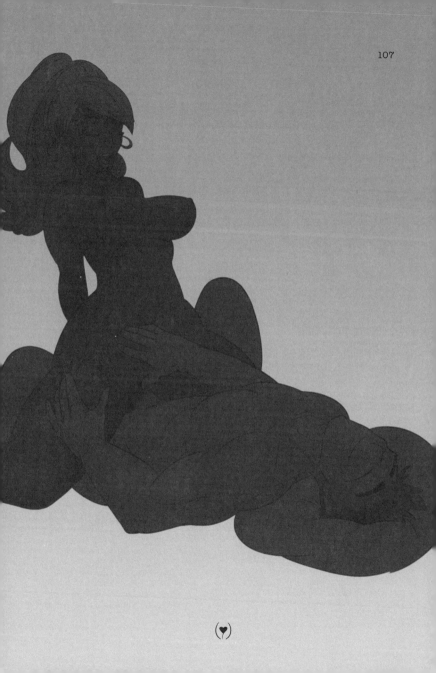

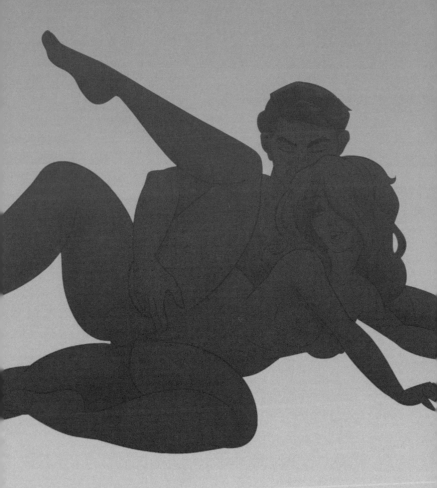

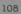

About Dr. Sadie

Dr. Sadie Allison, founder and CEO of Tickle Kitty, Inc., is author and publisher of today's most popular line of fun, informative, how-to sex-help books—the kind you wish you'd read earlier in life.

As a leading authority on human sexuality for over a decade, Dr. Sadie's mission is to empower women and men to embrace a deeper enjoyment of their sexuality, through encouragement, accurate information and inspiration. Her bestselling books include *Tickle His Pickle, Ride 'Em Cowgirl!, Tickle Your Fancy, TOYGASMS!* and *Tickle My Tush.* Each has won the coveted Independent Publisher's Best Sexuality Book Award and together have sold more than two million copies.

Dr. Sadie appears regularly on TV and radio, including *Tyra, E!, Discovery Health, PlayboyTV,* and *Howard Stern.* She's a sought-after speaker and in 2013 delivered her prestigious TEDx Talk called *Fearless Giving.* Dr. Sadie is also quoted regularly in *Cosmopolitan, Redbook, Men's Health* and WebMD.

Dr. Sadie earned her Doctorate from the Institute for Advanced Study of Human Sexuality and is a member of the American Association of Sex Educators, Counselors & Therapists (AASECT).

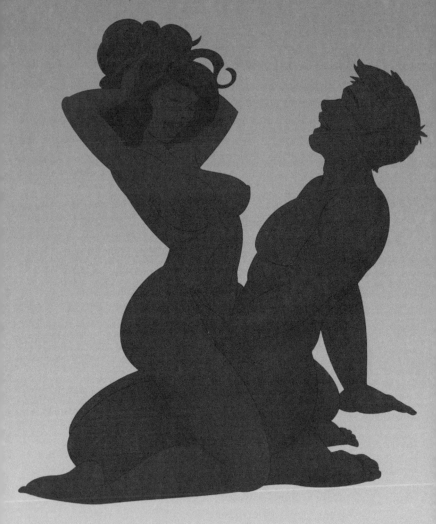

Special Thanks!

To my all-star publishing team for another outstanding book: J. Crocker Norge, Andrew Wislocki, Daniel Chan, Todd Gallopo, and Reid Mihalko. You make me shine.

And to my incredible family—your love and loyal support mean the world to me.

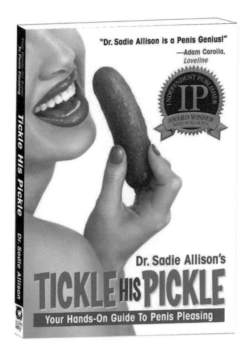

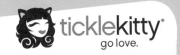
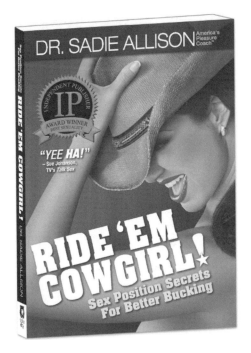

The Pleasure You Seek Is Right Behind You!

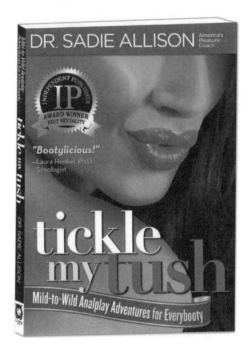

Tickle My Tush
Mild-to-Wild Analplay Adventures for Everybooty

Discover exciting new passions with the word's most fun and accessible how-to buttplay guide—comfortably, pleasurably and at your own pace.

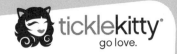

Pleasure at Your Fingertips!

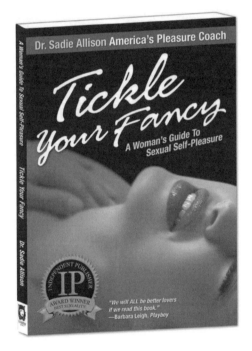

Tickle Your Fancy
A Woman's Guide to Sexual Self-Pleasure

A gentle and empowering guide to self-love
and orgasms for women—and the
"other team's playbook" for men.

Unleash Your Wildest Orgasms Ever!

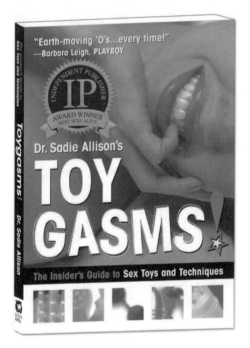

TOYGASMS!
The Insider's Guide to Sex Toys and Techniques

Explore the shapes, sizes and sensations that'll satisfy
you and your lover—along with stimulating ways
to achieve the strongest orgasms yet!

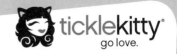
ticklekitty®
go love.

Glide into Slippery Bliss!

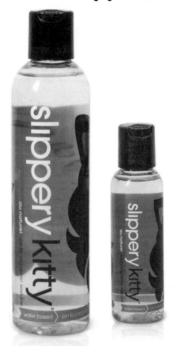

Slippery Kitty Lubricants
Au Naturel & Strawberry • 2 oz. & 8 oz.

Specially formulated by Dr. Sadie. Water-based, pH
balanced, paraben- and glycerin-free, condom compatible,
long-lasting and enriched with Aloe Vera & Vitamin E.

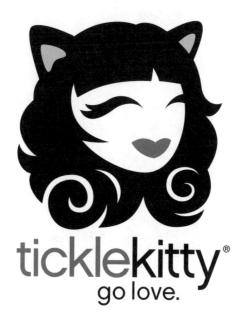

tickle**kitty**®
go love.

Tickle Kitty, Inc.
San Francisco, CA U.S.A.
TickleKitty.com